Kids Eat

A quick guide to getting your kids to eat nutritious food

By Melissa D. McPheeters

DEDICATION

This book is dedicated to my husband and children. Thank you for being my unwitting guinea pigs for the recipes I try. You inspired this book and you inspire me. I cook for you and feed you nutritious food because I'm selfish. I want you around me for as long as possible. I will continue to stuff your faces full of good food for as long as I live....and I'll make sure there are plenty of left overs in the fridge when I die.

Table of Contents

INTRODUCTION

They say necessity is the mother of all inventions. I always thought that was limited to physical inventions, like the television. That was most definitely invented by a dad who just needed to have something to entertain his kids, while he read the paper in peace. The woman who invented the boxed wine, I'm assuming is a woman who has kids, and just needed the convenience of an easy to pour wine that sits in the fridge, without the guilt of seeing just how much she is drinking. Apparently, I have invented a way to get kids to eat healthy. At least that's what I'm told. Honestly, my path to my children eating healthy was sheer stupidity on my part. Use my stupidity to your advantage.

Often, and I mean really often, I get asked by other moms what my secret is to get my kids to eat so healthy. It seems like common sense because the answer is simple. I just give it to them. There you go, you can put down the book and get back to your boxed wine.

Oh. You are still here. Ok. Let's get into it.

In the last five years or so, I became interested in how food plays a role in our overall health. Prior to that, I only cared about which foods would make me fat. I would religiously buy those stupid 100 calorie packs of processed junk, thinking it was healthy for me. I grew up on fast food, TV dinners and canned chili by the gallon from PriceClub (now it's called Costco). Not sure why my mom had an affinity for a flat of Stagg Chili, but she did, and we ate it. Whenever we would eat a veggie, it was always from the can. There is not enough butter in the world that can make canned veggies taste good. Blah!

I definitely didn't set out to make sure my kids eat super healthy. In fact, when I was pregnant, I didn't care too much about eating healthy for my baby. I mean, I pretended to care. I'm not a monster. I know, I sound like a horrible mother, and you're probably thinking the hospital should have kept my kids. Perhaps. I was fairly convinced my first child was going to come out a burrito instead of a baby. I ate bean burritos from Taco Bell more often than I would care to admit. With my second child, it was donuts, all day every day. With my third, more bean and cheese burritos. Now, even though I'm a disgusting human being when I'm pregnant, I actually do like to eat nutritious foods when I'm not pregnant. I feel like we only have this one body to get us through life, and I want to take care of it. I want to pass that on to my kids, so when they are in old age, they are healthy and happy, not sick, on bed rest, and a million doctor visits with just as many pills to pop.

HOW IT STARTED

The best place to start is from the beginning. If you already have kids with craptastic eating habits, stick with me as I have tips for you, too. When I was pregnant with my first child, we were so poor, we had no business having a kid, but life is like a Nike commercial and you just do it. During this time my husband was smack-dab in the middle of a mid-life crisis, quitting his job to become an actor. You read that right, an actor. Here we were broke, unemployed, and expecting our first bundle of joy. You know what is super expensive? Formula. That shit must have some gold in it. Needless to say, we couldn't afford formula, and I couldn't squirrel away enough free samples to feed my kid on a consistent basis. I had no choice but to breastfeed my kid. On that unforgettable day that he was born, I looked him in his sweet, little, bleary newborn eyes and told him, "You nurse, or you starve! We can't afford formula to feed you. I really like you and hope you stick with me." Thankfully, for all involved, he nursed.

Once I mastered nursing, and felt comfortable that I could keep my kid alive, it was time to introduce solid food. I was freaking out.

Those jars of baby food are expensive. Like $1.79 a jar. And to think he would need several jars a day! I was doing the math, and again, couldn't afford it. I did what any self-respecting mom would do, and I hit up my boyfriend, Google, for some advice. Turns out you can make your own baby food. It's just puréed fruit and veggies. Are you hearing me? There is a business based on puréeing food so babies can eat it! You are perfectly capable of puréeing. I promise.

This was around my birthday, so I hit up my mother in law for an immersion blender and got down to business. There is a pretty great website called *WholesomeBabyFood.com* that I used to help me learn how to prepare the food. Here I am with a baby who has only eaten fresh, whole, unprocessed food. You know what they put in store-bought baby food? Preservatives! I think preservatives taste gross. Carrots don't taste like carrots and apples taste weird. How can we expect our kids to like nutritious foods when the food we have been feeding them their whole lives doesn't taste right? My kids love to get those little fruit pouches at birthday parties. The packaging is enticing to them with all the fun colors. They always take one sip and put it down. My kids aren't used to the preservative taste and don't want to eat it. Just the other day, my 6 month old proved this point again. He has had fresh, puréed apples for a few weeks, at this point. We were traveling and after a long day on the road, we ended up at a fast food joint. I was being lazy and didn't want to dig his food out of the back of my fully packed SUV. Judge me all you want, but I was on the road for 7 hours with three kids, by myself, for what was suppose to be a two and a half hour drive. I'm just keeping it real with you. I ordered him some applesauce from the menu. He took two bites and then refused to eat the rest. I looked on the label and not only did it have preservatives in it but also High Fructose Corn Syrup. I'm fairly proud that my little man's palate wouldn't tolerate junk.

It's not like my kids have never had fast food or just crap food. They have and they love it. When I was pregnant with my third baby, my older two lived off of Happy Meals, hot dogs and PB&J's. I'm not proud of it, but it's a fact. The thing is, if kids have a choice, they will always choose the crap food. It's up to us as their parents to fill our house with nutritious foods. My kids will always choose Oreo's over apples. Guess who doesn't buy Oreos? This bitch. I'm not into fighting with my kids. They fight enough as it is. You know what else I don't buy for my kids? Juice boxes and soda. My kids drink water and milk. That's it. Juice boxes are for parties; they don't belong in your home. The only reason we have soda in my house is because I can't drink my whiskey straight. I'm no Carrie Underwood. My kids know that soda is for adults, like alcohol. Recently, my oldest was sitting next to a friend that was asking her dad for Coke-a-Cola. Without any hesitation my kid jumped into the conversation and told his friend that "Soda is junk food; it's bad for your body!" On the outside I was calm, cool, collected. On the inside, I was fist pumping like a cast member of *Jersey Shore.*

Melissa D. McPheeters

FOOD

I hear a lot of debate about organic food, especially when you should buy it, when it doesn't matter, etc. I don't buy organic produce. I don't have that kind of money to burn. We eat a shit ton of produce and organic is just out of the question for us. I'm also of the mind that if bugs can adapt and become resistant to the pesticides, then human beings can tolerate the small amount we ingest. I'm also assuming that all humans do as I do and wash their fruits and vegetables before eating them. That being said, if you can afford to buy organic produce, I think it's smart. We really don't know what Monsanto is up to, and I don't like them, or anyone playing God with our food supply. I do buy organic animal products. Organic milk, turkey, chicken and eggs are all staples in our home. It's more of a moral thing than a health thing. I think all animals need to be treated humanely, and the organic stamp is typically indicative of that. Not always, but it's a start. Also, since organic animal products are expensive as fuck, it helps me to eat a more plant-based diet. Remember, we the poor people.

A few documentaries have helped shaped my views on food as

a whole. *Food Inc., Fat Sick and Nearly Dead PT 1 and 2, Super Juice Me, and Fed Up.* There is also a good Netflix series called *Rotten.* Now, some of these have an agenda and propaganda, but you are smart and can sort that shit out.

I also like food that spoils. Not rotten food, but food that needs to be in the fridge. Now this is the thing with food that spoils: you need to prep it, or have it within eye sight. There is nothing worse than changing out your wine box to find a rotten cantaloupe behind it. Put everything at eye level. If you have peaches getting too ripe on the counter, put them in a bowl in the fridge so your kids see it when they open the fridge. I highly encourage you to prep food because it makes those busy days that much more manageable. Also, adults and kids can be funny about just how they like their food served. I won't ever eat a whole apple, but I'll chow down on apple slices. Find out how your kids like things and do it.

I don't make my kids eat gross food, either. No kale here. Fuck kale. I once made my boss leave a café since everything on their menu had kale in it. We went to Roscoe's Chicken and Waffles instead. It was divine.

PUT IT ON THEIR PLATE

One of the most important things you can do in your quest to have your kids eat healthy is to live it. You can't expect your kids to want pineapple for a snack if you are sitting there with a bag of potato chips. I heard somewhere that kids will do as you do, not as you say. So be the example. I know that I'm a big, fat hypocrite with the whole soda for my whiskey thing. I accept that and any judgement.

I'm not here to judge you on what you choose to feed your kids. If you want to feed them Burger King every day, more power to you. Just don't complain to me that your kids will only eat junk. If you want them to eat healthy, hear me when I say: *just put it on their plate*. It's as simple as that. I never make a different meal for my kids than what my husband and I are eating. What I have done is deconstruct our meal. Say we are having chicken burrito bowls for dinner. I will separate out the rice, beans, chicken, avocado, cheese, whatever. Kids can be funny when everything is piled on each other. At least my kids can be. This way they see each food and understand that this is the food we eat. I never ask them if they want what we are having. They will always say no. I just put it on their plate. Have you ever asked a 6 month old if he wants what you are about to give him? No. Don't start now.

When they were toddlers, I would always put one thing I knew they liked on their plate and two or three things that we were eating. They see the food and know it's normal, etc. Sometimes they would try it and other times they would ignore it. What if they don't eat it, you say! I don't want to waste food, you say! There are starving children in Africa, you say! I say don't put as much food on *your* plate. You eat what they don't. Food doesn't go to waste and you are modeling the behavior. Win. Win.

THE DAMAGING NARRATIVE

S top saying that your kid is a picky eater or that your kid will only eat this one thing. Not true. You are creating and carrying on a narrative. Knock it off. I have never once said my kids are picky eaters, even when they won't eat what I just spent an hour cooking. I chalk it up to the fact that they just don't feel like eating whatever we are having. They are human, after all. My oldest recently had a phase where he would yell when I placed his dinner in front of him, "I'm not eating this! This is disgusting!" All before the kid even tried it. Did I say, "Ok. I'll make you an Oreo and candy sandwich instead?" No. Fuck no. I'm the mom. I told him he didn't have to eat it all, but he did need to try it. Nine times out of ten he will take a bite, give me the thumbs up, and tell me "I like your *cook*, Mom!" I also remind my kids that I'm not making them something gross. I have to eat it, too.

I have a wonderful mom-friend who swears her kid is a picky eater. She is always shocked when he is at my house devouring apple slices. Well, except the skin. He is apparently offended by the skin. Maybe it's a texture thing? Don't know. She is so adamant that her kid is a picky eater that she brought a separate meal for him when I had them over for dinner. See, she is super mom! I would never bring a secondary meal because I'm lazy as all get out. Fast forward to dinner time and all the kids are sitting around the kiddie table happily eating the meal I had prepared. She is shocked and can't believe her kid is eating what I put on his plate. This is part peer pressure (more on peer pressure later) and part just putting it on his plate. Just then, the oven timer goes off. She opens the oven to reveal the chicken nuggets she brought for her kid. All the kids see the glorious, golden nuggets and abandon the meal they were happily eating. Now everyone is screaming about NUGGETS!!!! My point is, if kids have a choice, they will always choose the crap food. Except for my six-month old. He is too special of a human being.

You say your kid will only eat one thing. You are a dirty rotten liar. Your kid just has your number and is playing you. What this is really about is that you don't want to deal with a tantrum. I get it, neither do I. But you are the parent. Not them. If you let them have control now, you better buckle up for their teenage years. Kids need nutrients from a variety of sources. It's not healthy to only eat chips or tortillas or yogurt. What will they eat, you say? They will starve, you say! I say, Mom and Dad the fuck up. Kids are human beings. As human beings we have a natural instinct to survive. Number one on the survival front is eating. Just put it on their plate. They will scream, they will yell, and they will eventually eat.

Please, stop telling kids to eat when you are at the dinner table. They know what to do when they have a plate of food in front of them. They aren't idiots. Well, some are, but I'll get to that later. I cringe every time I hear an adult badger a kid to "Eat your veggies, little Timmy. Eat. EAT. EAT!!!!!" If you were getting bitched at every time you sat down to eat, that wouldn't make it a place you would want to be. You need to shut up. What I do suggest you talk about is the different foods that are on the plate. How to eat them, where they came from, different ways you can cook them, why you like them. Kids are fascinated with that shit. You know what they don't give a shit about? Growing up big and strong. That's some far off notion and they don't care. They do seem to care about staying healthy. We eat nutritious foods so we can stay healthy. We exercise to stay strong. That is here and now; they get it.

Melissa D. McPheeters

LEARN TO COOK

This brings me to another, important topic. Learn how to cook. It's really not that hard. We have the internet. It's full of all these recipes, which are literally instructions, step by step, on how to make something. They also have a convenient star system to let you know other people like it. Get yourself a set of decent knives, a knife sharpener thing, and get to chopping. Prep as much as you can and leave it eyelevel in the fridge. You and your kids will be more inclined to eat healthy if it's convenient. Watermelon, strawberries, bell peppers, carrots, celery, cucumbers, and pineapple are all easily prep-able. Yes, it's annoying and time consuming to chop up all those fruits and veggies. But it's worth it. And, if you are wealthy, you can always buy the precut packages of fruits and veggies at the market. I'm not, so I chop.

There is this thing that is kind of funny to humans. We like one thing prepared a certain way but won't eat the same thing prepared another way. I am not the biggest fan of tomatoes. I'll usually eat around them or pick them out. However, I devour salsa. I think my insides are 50% salsa and 50% whiskey. I cannot get enough salsa….and salsa is primarily tomatoes. My oldest isn't the biggest fan of large zucchini chunks, but loves it in the meatballs I make. If your kid doesn't like something, try making it another way. I don't like raw broccoli unless its smothered in ranch dressing, but I love cooked broccoli with onions and garlic.

Another excuse I hear about eating healthy is that it's expensive. No. It is not. You can buy 10 apples for the same amount of money as a bag of Doritos. It will take you longer to eat the apples than the bag of chips. I have a mom friend who told me she spends $400 a week on groceries. A week! That is insane to me. I spend $150. I go to two different stores to get the best value. Produce is from Sprouts since I like the quality and they have the best prices. Pantry staples are from Vons because they are typically on sale there. Also, once a month I hit up Costco for their organic turkey, eggs, milk and chicken, since it's more cost effective. Yes, it takes time to go to three different places, but eventually you get in a rhythm and you can expedite things. You know what also takes a lot of time? Going to the doctor since you filled your body with crap and now it's revolting or standing in line at the pharmacy to get all your prescriptions because you aren't fueling your body properly. It's our job as parents to set our kids up for life as an adult. I will take the time now to make sure they are healthy so they don't have to take the time later.

I don't think meals need to be super fancy, either. They just need to include the basics: fruits, veggies, protein and a starch. I am a firm believer that brown rice, black beans, and avocado is a perfectly acceptable meal. Turkey, cheese and strawberries make a fine lunch. Don't make yourself crazy.

MEAL PLANNING

In the last few years I have gotten into meal planning. I set aside some time and write down what we will have for dinner each night of the week. I can plan for the days I know we won't be home for dinner and the days I work late. I'm looking at you, Crock Pot, you sexy thing. My husband takes the left overs for lunch the next day. It saves a ton of time and money since it stops the "What do you want for dinner?" game, which always results in ordering pizza or eating cereal. My list is pretty fluid, since life can get in the way of the best laid plan. I might not have the Zucchini Meatballs tonight since I forgot to defrost the turkey, but I'll have them tomorrow, and make what I was going to make tomorrow today. We all know that if you shop from a list that you will save time and money since you aren't aimlessly meandering around the market and buying impulsively.

Melissa D. McPheeters

DON'T BUY IT

S eems like a simple enough concept, but yet I see over and over parents buying junk for their kids while complaining that their kids eat junk. Stop buying it! Seriously. If your kid will only eat Happy Meals, then stop going to McDonalds. It's not like your kid has a car, a license, and cash, much less knows how to get to McDonalds. Stop it. If your kid will only eat Pringles, stop buying the Pringles. My middle child has a love affair with those little yogurts. Not the tubes, but the little smoothie type ones with the fun characters on it, the ones with a shit ton of sugar. She couldn't say yogurt so she called them "Ya Ya's". Well, she would freak out in order to have a Ya Ya. She would demand them all the time. Three AM, time for a Ya Ya. In the bath tub, Ya Ya time! She has an imaginary scratch on her foot from her imaginary nemesis, only a Ya Ya will do. Like a moron, I would buy them time and time again. I figured I want my daughter to like me, and she likes me because I buy her these sugar laden Ya Ya's. No. Wrong. She likes me because I taught her to use the toilet and not shit in her pants. She likes me because I cuddle her at night when she is scared and wipe the tears from her face after she walks into a wall for the millionth time. Guess what I finally did? I stopped buying them. She had a tantrum and then got over it. Your kid will too.

INCLUDE THEM

A big reason why kids won't eat what you want them to is it's a control thing. Let them have control. My Ya Ya loving middle child loves to peruse the produce section with me. We talk about the different fruits and veggies, how they taste, how you cook them, etc. We find new things and bring them home for the whole family to try. This is how we discovered Dinosaur Egg Pluots, which led to a bigger conversation on what is a pluot. A pluot is a plum and an apricot. This led to an interest in trying a plum and an apricot independently. Give them control when you can.

I've read some advice advocating for your kids to help you in the kitchen. I say hell no. Just because I'm lazy and am trying to hold my shit together and can't possibly add one more thing, like keeping them safe, while I'm putting together dinner. Plus, when I'm cooking, it's my time with my other boyfriend, Jack Daniels. But seriously, if you can muster the patience to have your kids help put meals together, I think that it would only increase their interest in trying nutritious foods, provided you aren't deep frying Oreo's.

Melissa D. McPheeters

RULES FOR THE TABLE

W e don't have too many rules for the dinner table. My biggest one that I enforce like a savage beast is no feet on the table. Other than that, it's pretty relaxed at my table. We don't allow tablets or phones, as we like to actually converse with each other. Our kids don't have to eat everything that is on their plate. They just need to try it. Obviously if there is something in particular that I know my kid hates, I don't bother putting it on her plate. The only thing that I've come across that they just can't get on board with is shrimp. I've tried it several ways and it's just a no go for them.

Surprisingly I'm ok with my kids snacking up until meal time. I'm not into having crazy kids at the table because they are so hungry. When my kids are hungry, they are incredibly unreasonable. I give zero shits about spoiling their appetite. If they want to snack on blueberries up until I'm literally plating their food, fine by me. Once dinner is on the table, snacking stops and they are expected to eat or try what is on their plate. I just know to not put as much food on their plate, so as to not waste food, and we have more left-overs for the next day. This might be why they are fairly open to trying new things. Their bodies aren't ravenous so they are more amenable to eating what's on their plate.

USE THINGS TO YOUR ADVANTAGE

At some point my kid got interested in death. It's a weird concept for them, and an even weirder one to explain without totally terrorizing them. When my oldest was four, he became very interested in how and where he would die. Despite my reassurance that it was a long way off, he kept peppering me with questions. One morning while we were getting him ready for preschool he asked if he would die on the toilet. Like the great mother that I am I said, "No. But do you know who did die on the toilet? Elvis." Then I proceeded to takes some liberties and told him how Elvis wasn't eating a healthy diet and that is why he died on the toilet. Which also led to a slightly embarrassing conversation with his preschool teacher, as he was concerned that snack time wouldn't be healthy, landing him dead on the toilet.

The great thing about Elvis and the toilet is that it turned into an ongoing conversation on what is and isn't healthy to eat. We came up with a point system to help him figure out what is healthy.

One is total junk and 10 is healthy. For the next year he had me rating the food he was about to eat. Not once did our point system keep him from eating something in the 1-4 range. What it did do was make him aware of what he was eating and we had some great conversations about nutrition.   My point is, use these situations to your advantage. Take some liberties and make it work.

PEER PRESSURE

U nder the subject of using things to your advantage is Peer Pressure. It can be a bitch, but you can also work it in your favor. I have a wonderful mom friend who swears that her kid will only eat donuts and Pringles. They come over for play dates often and she is shocked to see her kid eating watermelon. Her kid is eating it because my kids are eating it. Peer Pressure.

So here you are, you've been putting the healthy food on their plates, but they haven't touched it. You've eaten it and have been more regular than you have been in years. Now what? You go and plan a play date with that mom who feeds her kids kale chips and seaweed. You know the one I'm talking about. Make sure it's at her house, too. Snack time comes, she offers a healthy snack. She is a take it or leave it kind of mom. So retro. I love her. Your child takes it and eats it. You are picking your jaw up off the floor. Your kid is eating it because she has seen the food before since you've been putting it on her plate, and because her friend is happily eating it. Peer Pressure. Use it to your advantage.

The kind of peer pressure I want you to avoid is other Sanctimommies, the ones who *could* never, *would* never, do exactly whatever it is that you are doing right now. Recently, I was in my kid's school during snack time. The snack mom was droning on about how the apple slices she so thoughtfully sliced had turned brown by the time snack came around. I offered up a quick tip: if you put the slices in a bowl of salt water for a minute and then rinse, they won't turn brown. I shit you not, it was like I suggested we dip the apples in meth. She said, "I could *never* give children *this* small *salt!*" Not sure if she knows that human beings, big and small, need some salt to live. I was more annoyed that she just pumped my kid full of sugar with her homemade banana bread and now has the audacity to get all high and mighty over a mineral. Avoid these people if you can, and if you can't just take what they have to say with a grain of salt.

TREATS

U gh. Treats. I don't say this because I don't like them or think my kids shouldn't enjoy them now and then. I typically don't keep them in my house as, like I said, I'm not into fighting with my kids. My big problem is when other people surprise my kids with treats. It's a Pandora's box. Typically, you will get people who want to treat your kids with a box of crazy candy or chocolate, giving it to them right before lunch, or worse, bed time. Then you, as the parent, are stuck in this vortex of what to do. If you say no, then you are in the middle of a tantrum and the fallen face of the gifter. If you say yes, then you are in a special brand of hell that only other parents can appreciate. Most people who give your kids treats are people who don't have kids. People who have kids give you Amazon gift cards. They know. Now, I've been in a situation or two when someone has wanted to gift my kids total crap and I've had to be the bad guy. You know what? I don't care. If you want to spend the next hour with my kids all high on sugar, be my guest. But I don't. I sure as shit am not going to allow you to drop a sugar bomb and walk away. It has led to some awkward conversations with loved ones, but it's typically more awkward for them than me. One-time offenders I let slide, but if you continually bring my kids crap under the guise that you are treating them, well, we will have a conversation to put a stop to it.

Believe it or not, I would like to be the one treating my kids. It's exhausting always making sure that my kids are being fed nutritious foods, planning meals, etc. I want to be the "good guy" once in a while. This is why I devised the "Donut Date." It's exactly what it sounds like. Every few months I take my kids to get a donut and milk. We sit in the donut shop and talk about our day. It's awesome. Since it doesn't happen too often it really helps drive home the point of a treat. We all look forward to it, and it is super fun.

Halloween is one of my favorite holidays, if not *the* favorite. Not because of the candy, but because of the decorations, costumes and parties we throw every year. I came to a sort of crossroad on how to handle the influx of candy. My kids definitely don't need three pounds of candy coursing through their tiny bodies. However, they worked damn hard pounding the pavement to get the candy. My mom told me of an idea she saw online: trade candy for a toy. A few years ago I gave it a whirl, to much success. My kids have 24 hours with their candy and then I offer them a coveted toy to trade it for. Last year my oldest was on to me. He told me that he didn't want to trade his candy. Fair enough. I bought the toy any way. Twenty-four hours pass, and I offer the trade. Sure as shit, he traded. This year my kid already had a toy in mind that he wanted to trade for. I get that lots of parents won't agree with me on this tactic. However, for me, it beats dealing with kids on a sugar high. I'm just not into it.

SNACK BAG

The biggest tool you can have in your quest for healthy eaters is the Snack Bag. Before you scrunch up your nose at how much work this sounds like, hear me out. It is a lot of work, but it's worth it. Now we have all been there when our kids are freaking out in the back seat because they are hungry and we end up at the pretzel stand spending $25 on bread. The snack bag puts an end to this madness. I always pack a snack bag when we go out. Pack more than you know they will ever eat. The snack bag typically consists of 5 different fruits and veggies, a protein, and a starch. Excessive? Yes. But it works. Also, I make sure to double it up. I put two of everything in it so my kids don't fight. Like I said, I'm not into them fighting as much as they are into fighting with themselves.

Go get yourself an insulated lunch box from your big box retailer or Amazon. Make sure you get one with a character your kids like on it. Remember: you have to romance them, you need to make it enticing. While you are at it, get one of those slim ice packs. I like the Bento ones. They are imperative. No one likes warm cucumber.

This is why the snack bag works so well: You fill it with all the healthy food you want your kids to eat. They freak out in the car or park or wherever because they are "starving!!!". Hand them the snack bag and they feel like masters of their universe since they get to decide what to eat. They get to choose from what you deem healthy. It's genius and it works. Anything that my kids don't eat I put in the fridge for the snack bag the next day, or I eat it while I'm watching *Real Housewives*. Nothing goes to waste.

When my eldest started Kindergarten I made him the most epic snack bag for school. Just my humble opinion. My Ya Ya loving middle child insisted that I make her a special snack bag, too. I tried reasoning with a two-year old, as she wasn't going to school and didn't need a snack bag. I am smart like that. Well, after a huge tantrum, I acquiesced to her demand and made her a snack bag. Turns out that you should absolutely listen to a two-year old once in a while. Having the snack bags prepped in the morning cuts down on my time in the kitchen the rest of the day. Whenever they want another snack, I just point them to their bag. It's perfection.

KIDS ARE DUMB

Not really, but they can be. Don't assume that your kid knows how to eat watermelon. Seems like common sense, but it's not. I know this sweet-faced kid who refuses to eat fruits or veggies. One day his mom was badgering him to eat some watermelon since he was having poop issues. He finally caved and took a slice. I'm sitting across from him and watched him try to take a bite out of the rind! It's no wonder he thinks watermelon is gross. I taught him how to eat the watermelon and explained to him that with some fruits and veggies you only eat the inside, not the skin. Now the kid loves watermelon.

My husband told me about a time that he had his sweet 90-year old grandma at his condo. She is one of the best ladies I have ever met, one of those people that you just wish you had more time with. He was cutting up some red bell pepper and offered her a slice. She declined, stating that she couldn't eat anything spicy. My husband gently told her that they are actually sweet. She tried it and loved it. She couldn't believe she went ninety years avoiding them!

Melissa D. McPheeters

IT'S UP TO YOU

This whole "eating healthy" thing is up to you. Make it a priority and it will happen. Purée your baby food; avoid processed food with preservatives. Put the foods you want your kids to eat on their plates. Stop the narrative you have going on, and don't live in your excuses. Live the lifestyle you want your kids to live. Learn to cook. Use things to your advantage. Manage treats as you see fit. Get yourself a snack bag. Teach your kids. Above all, you can do this. We only have this one life, so just do your best.

Go slow. If this is a complete overhaul for you, just drop one bad thing and add one good thing every time you shop. Before you know it, your house will be stocked full of the nutritious foods you want, and depleted of the crap food you don't.

I'm not a doctor, nutritionist, healer, or anything like that. I'm just a mom who stumbled upon a way to get my kids to eat nutritious foods. We are too poor to go out to eat very often, so when we do, I let my kids eat whatever they want. The feeling is, at home we have and eat only nutritious foods, but when we are out, we splurge. That idea doesn't work if you go out to eat for every meal. Use common sense, and remember, your kids are humans, too. Being kind to them includes building healthy habits, not just giving in to their demands of cookies and churros. Come to think of it, churros *are* delicious.